A Foreign Nurse's Guide to America

A Foreign Nurse's Guide to America

SHIRLEY LORRAINE FRANKS, RN, BS, MBA

iUniverse, Inc.
Bloomington

A FOREIGN NURSE'S GUIDE TO AMERICA

iUniverse books may be ordered through booksellers or by contacting:

iUniverse
1663 Liberty Drive
Bloomington, IN 47403
www.iuniverse.com
1-800-Authors (1-800-288-4677)

ISBN: 978-1-4697-3817-8 (sc)
ISBN: 978-1-4697-3819-2 (hc)
ISBN: 978-1-4697-3818-5 (ebk)

Printed in the United States of America

iUniverse rev. date: 02/02/2012

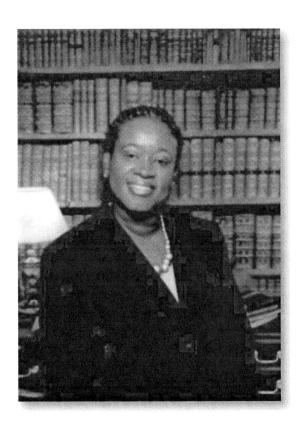

Shirley Lorraine Franks, RN, BS, MBA

Contents

Acknowledgements

To my mother, Girlie Franks, who taught me how to read and love books at early age in life.

To Dale Morton, a mutual friend, and an alumni of University of the Virgin Islands—and still an employee at the University of the Virgin Islands—thanks for being an inspiration to me from the beginning of my college years.

To my children Sai and Harmonii—who are the rock and love of my life.

To all those who supported me in the motivation and inspiration toward the completion of this book, including Pastor Joel Osteen, the late Jim Rohn, and Matthew Barnett, author of "*The Cause Within You*", and Phil Munsey, author of a "*Legacy Now*".

To my dear friend and colleague, Dr. George E. Griffin, thanks for your words of encouragement and for being an awesome influence in my life. He has provided great inspiration and professional support to me for many years.

Preface

I GRADUATED *CUM LADE* FROM the nursing program in St. Thomas, United States, Virgin Islands. I give my thanks to Dr. Maxine Nunez, Registered Nurse, PhD of the nursing program then. A native of St. Thomas, Maxine Nunez was my mentor. She guided me from the start of the program to finish. She was very shrewd but kind. In the meantime, I tested out and successfully passed anatomy, and physiology. As a biology lover, it was not a great I think that Maxine Nunez had the confidence in me. I successfully passed and obtained eight credits that were applied to the nursing program. I was given a two-year plot and I followed it. I took 18.5 credits each semester and nine credits during the summer. I started the nursing program in August 1981 and graduated in May 1983. I did the National Council Licensure Examination (NCLEX) and successfully passed the examination.in May; I started working as a graduate nurse at Roy Schneider hospital in Charlotte Amalie, St. Thomas. I was enrolled in the Associate Diploma Nursing (ADN) program. Upon graduation, I successfully had completed 89 credit hours. I was successful at Nursing Board Examination and became a Registered Nurse (RN) in July 1983. I was a good student. To be successful, the late Jim Rohn said that one must be a good student. I listened to my mentor and followed instructions. After two years of work at the hospital, I relocated to the United States mainland where I still reside. I give honor to my mother, Girlie Franks, who financially provided during my college years. I am still a student, currently pursuing a Master Degree in Nursing. I possess a Master's Degree in Business Association (MBA) and may attain a PhD in nursing one day.

In May 1985, I worked as an Emergency Department (ED) Nurse at Roy Schneider's Hospital in St. Thomas. My nursing experience was wonderful. We worked closely with the paramedics. Many of the ED nurses were locally trained nurses; others were from Canada, or the United States mainland. The foreign nurses there were mostly from contracted nursing agencies. We welcome them. The nursing environment was a team collaborative approach. There was no Licensed Professional Nurses (LPN's) working the ED. Many of the physicians were from on islands. It was a 12-bed Emergency Room, including a cardiac and a trauma room. What I loved about my experience there at hospital, was the camaraderie involved with the paramedics. The paramedics were stationed at the ED. We worked eight-hour shifts. The learning experience was intensive. I wanted more. I wanted to explore other horizons.

In 1985, I turned in my resignation to my Supervisor. The reason I gave was that I relocating to the United States to further my education. Deep down it was actually to explore an excitement trip in my nursing career. My emotions were stirred in the pursuit of nursing to exploit nursing in the mainland. I wished to explore what was on the other side, so to speak. I set up for a nursing interview in Long Island at the Long Island College Hospital (LICH). I wanted to work in the Emergency Department (ED) because I was already an ED nurse in St. Thomas. I also loved the action. When I arrived in New York, the position offered to me was Telemetry nursing. I declined that position after I was called by a major trauma center. After that interview, I was offered an attractive position then to work in a large trauma center in New York City. Wow! I went back to the Virgin Islands. My phone kept ringing asking for a start date. Somewhat reluctantly, I turned my resignation on a mission to explore nursing the United States mainland, especially New York City.

New York was intriguing. I had family members there. It was a culture shock to say the least. I had to take three trains to get from Queens to Manhattan. It was at a teaching hospital. The experience was huge. I worked in the cardiac and trauma center. From stabbed wounds to gunshot wounds ... the excitement was real and thrilling. A code blue could be a young male that arrived by New York fire department with a heart rate of 250. Back then verapamil was the drug of choice. Now adenosine is now the drug of choice. We may have to cardiovert. It was exciting! The experience was awesome. Plus, I worked among a diverse culture of nurses. Nursing has since become even more diverse.

There was a nursing shortage. That was told to us (nurses) since then. We worked constantly in yellow disposable gowns because at that time Human Immunodeficiency Virus (HIV) was rapidly becoming an epidemic. Health care workers did not really know the cause and treatment was not as aggressive. If one is travelling the number two or number three train ... only God knows what one can encounter. Many of the travelers on the number two and number three were IV drug users. Sharing needles was not an option! Some were coming from stop houses or going back home or just sleeping on the train for the next stop. One day, I got off on the wrong stop. It was a Sunday. I was on 8th avenue instead of 6th avenue. The subway was quiet. I encountered a gang group dressed in black and white. Flight or fright! I took off running racing back to the train stop. Luckily one pulled up and I got on. It was the first discernment that I received regarding the reason I am here. I got to work safely, but I was late. As time went by, I was challenged by the travelling to and from work. It was a hassle. Shortly after I turned in my resignation and headed south.

Introduction

THE REASON IN WRITING A *Foreign Nurse's Guide To America* is to serve as a guide to foreign nurses as a preparation and to what that can be expected on their journey to America. I discovered that during my nursing journey here, there were misconceptions that I encountered. The major misconception focused on diversity. Diversity in healthcare and nursing are quite common. Some of us chuckle to some of the comments or misconception. However, my perception that a foreign nurse can be respected in the nursing field, if he or she were much more understood. To be understood, it is important that both parties understand diversification.

The book is written in a light version. It is easily readable.

The world is small now. The universe can be considered all around us. There are diverse cultures all over the world. However, I made discoveries to write A *foreign nurses Guide To America* to enlighten some of my colleagues. Additionally, one may decide whether a decision to relocate is feasible or not.

I gave an overview of my experience. From a nurse in the (United States Virgin Islands) USVI, I had a mission. I was mentored successfully, so I thought. I had to become a good student and like most nursing students we all had to be good students. Not everyone may have similar experiences. However, nursing students are usually well-guided. However, what is important is to be a good student. Making sure one is mentored properly is very important. As an experienced nurse with over 20 years' experience, I want to extend the following guide especially to foreign nurses:

- Establish a burning desire
- Set a goal
- Pursue that goal
- Avoid distractions
- Set a target educational goal
- Avoid procrastination
- Join a nurse membership in one's field, e.g., Emergency Nurses Association (ENA), or American Nurses' Association (ANA, for example.

Chapter One

My journey As A Nurse To The USA

I RELOCATED TO THE UNITED States mainland from St. Thomas, Virgin Islands in 1985. At that time, I worked as an Emergency room nurse. I went to the "Big Apple," New York City. I worked a big facility as an emergency room nurse. It was exciting. I completed by Bachelor's Degree. I have since then completed a Master's in Business Association (MBA). Currently, I am working on the completion of a Master's Degree in Nursing (MSN) with a concentration in Education. My plans are to complete a PhD in nursing.

I have gained vast experiences during my nursing journey here in the USA. I have learned tremendously. I have networked with from paramedics and nurses from all walks of life. In addition, to healthcare, I have acquired some business experiences in network marketing. I have also done travel nursing as well as hospital-based nursing.

During my experience, I have nurses asked me questions about how did I relocate to the US. I have also heard and observed others being confronted about such issues. Many nurses were unaware on the relocation process and may still be uninformed of the facts. Some nurses were not quite sure back then how reciprocity works.

Some were puzzled the reasons and rationale for relocation. There are questions as to why foreign nurses have left the exotic places such as the Caribbean and the Canada, for example, to relocate here to the USA. Times have changed. Hopefully it has. However, we reside in a diversified culture. The diversify culture is strongly seen in patients and healthcare workers. Some just did not get it all. Others were clueless regarding one's geographical location; others seemed concerned if one even knew how to practice nursing in the United States mainland. Sometimes I was puzzled myself regarding the questions that were thrown at you. In my mind, I kept thinking may be there should be a book or guide to educate other nurses. When I was in the Virgin Islands, I used to wonder why nurses would leave the United States mainland and come to Caribbean to work. Though their ability was never questioned; we welcome them. Most American travelled nurses would always work nights and spend days at the beach enjoying the sun and the Caribbean flavor. Many relocated from Canada as well. There were also nurses from the Philippines as well. In my experience, the relocated nurses were from the United States mainland, Canada, and the Philippines.

The nursing profession consists licensed professional nurses (LPN's) and Registered Nurses (RN's). The fundamentals stemmed on the nursing process. Florence Nightingale, the first nursing theorist, was born to She was the pioneer of nursing and was known as the" Lady with the Lamp" Florence was born in May 12 1820, in Florence, Italy (n.d. nightingale, 2011). She opened a nursing school in London. To this day, Florence is well recognized for her dedication to the nursing. National week is celebrated May 6-May 12 in honor of Florence Nightingale's birthday, May 12.

I have acquired a vast amount of experience and knowledge nursing my journey as a nurse. I relocated from the Virgin Islands several years ago to New York City. A conscious decision was made after two years of nursing experience in the Caribbean. I applied at a local hospital in Long Island and set up for an interview. The interview went well except I was offered a position as a Telemetry nurse. I was young and loved trauma nursing; also the hours were too long; they offered 10 hour and 12 hour shifts. I called a city hospital in New York City and got hired on the spot that same day. I went back to the Virgin Islands to resume my position temporarily. The nurse recruiter kept calling. Somewhat reluctantly, I submitted my resignation with plans to further my education in the United States. I was always in love with books, especially inspirational books. To this day, if my peers were to describe me I would be described as always seen reading a book or a magazine. I recognized that habit was developed from my mother. At the age of five, my mother gave me an encyclopedia as a birthday gift. My mother relocated from the island of St. Kitts and went to Curacao after my father died from a tragic accident. She herself travelled to many islands from the islands of St. Kitts-Nevis, the United States, Virgin Islands, Curacao, Puerto Rico, Florida, and New York. She has later retired in the Caribbean.

At age five, I thought I was a good reader. My games as a child was find it. My grandmother kept me as my mother traveled and worked. other siblings needs. Books that I have read as a child have pointed out to reflect what a person has done as a child creates was a passion for the child what your calling might be or what one's passion may be as adult. I remembered vividly childhood games played with my siblings and peers. My childhood games with my other cousins would be to read and find a book and find a word. The word will be selected from an inconspicuous place on the page while I counted in one's, fives, or tens. Whoever had the most words would win the game. My two favorite games would be to find it from reading and to sell. I would use my encyclopedia and read enhance my vocabulary. I would also practice how to read fast. Speed and accuracy were important. That was the purpose of find it words, reading a book. To this day it excites me. I have also taught my two children, Harmonii, and Sai to practice reading fast my doing that game.

Throughout my life I have read many books. I am a reader. I will go to bed with a book and wake up with a book. The late Jim Rohn, my most favorite author and philosopher, said *"leaders are readers"* (n.d. Jim Rohn). I have encouraged both my children to read at least 15 minutes per day. Both my children are excellent readers. Other authors who have influenced me are Anthony Robbins, Brian Tracy, Eckhart Tolle, Dale Carnegie, and Kevin Trudeau, and Zig Ziglar. Most of the books I read are business books, philosophical books, and inspirational books. Bibliography and history are important readings also. I am yet to incorporate more historical readings. In the past seven years, I very seldom look at television or read novels. Among important reading materials are bibliographies and histories of important people. I am not saying not to read novels; whatever one finds of interests is important favorable to them. My favorite magazines are *"Success" and "Travel Guide."*

As a child, I was obsessed with the idea of relocating to the United States before graduating from college, I remember a group of senior students gathered together to discuss plans. My plans were to relocate to the USA to practice nursing.

Before relocation, I worked in the ED at Roy Schneider's hospital as an Emergency nurse in St. Thomas. I had a one bedroom condo in St. Thomas. Life was great! I worked an eight hour shift. The commute was fine. The local bus transportation took about 15 minutes to arrive to work. Usually, I will walk home along the waterfront. This was my way of daily exercise. It was a casual walk, with the island breeze gently blowing into my face. Sometimes, I will stop at Palm Hotel located along the waterfront in Charlotte Amalie and treat myself to a Virgin Pina Colado. I remembered vividly consuming one Virgin Pina Colado then taking the other with me as I completed my journey home. For nurses who worked evening and night shifts, the hospital services provided transportation for those who needed it. If not, taxi services were reasonable, four dollars that I can remember. One major lunch was offered to all nurses free of charge. The cost price was $3.50. Anything over that cost were paid by the employee.

There were no real pressures to relocate. I wanted to explore life on the other side of the globe. I had relatives in New York. Throughout my existence here I kept asking myself why I really came here to the United States mainland. I left a beautiful island with friends and family; the working environment was great. I only realized it once I relocated here. We communicated well as nurses; the team spirit was excellent. The salary was not the same as the USA; however, when you compare the cost of living it may be turn out to be the same. Anthony Robbins says "do what you love." Donald Trump also said for one to do what one loves. In fact, most successful people would advise for one to do what one loves. It does not matter salary and living conditions, it is really about what one is happy with while helping others. Lifestyle is important; the true essence is happiness. Most people come to America seeking a better lifestyle; some seek true success because of unlimited opportunities that America has to over. Other reasons may not have been told, but it can be concluded about achieving "one's dream."

I love reading and writing. I also love to sell. While here in the United States. I have joined a few network marketing businesses

5

because of my quest for selling and helping others. I never told my up lines that I was a nurse for fear that they may not understand. Some people have asked why you are doing this when you are a nurse. Money is not always the objective of a business or one's career. Money may be a motivator; it is not about the money I would say. But when I look back as my childhood days, I would always be the seller when we play "family play." Go figure.

My mother also was a seller. She had a small shop. My mother funded my college fees. I did not owe any bills upon graduation. I give thanks and recognition to my mother and to God. Thanks Mom for the gift of an encyclopedia at age 4. Reading is one of my favorite hobbies.

Success must be sought after. It does not come by luck. Whatever one's religion, one should keep God's teaching in one's life. The Bible is a book that teachings us balance and God's word. We all need a balance. That balance includes a spiritual lifestyle. The late Jim Rohn recommended the Bible as a valuable teaching. One does not have to be a religious fanatic to read the bible.

In 1999, I was traveling on a nursing assignment to Nevada and while at the airport, I reflected on my life as a nurse. I pondered my reasons for here in the United States. I had my journal with me. In my journal I wrote a foreign nurse's guide to America. I made reflections myself I of the title *A Foreign Nurse's Guide To America*. An interested title to a book that could be a best seller, I thought. Yes! To this day as I write this book several years later, I am thanking God in advance for making "*A foreign Nurses' Guide*" to be a successful book seller and for also putting the vision in my mind. I am going to write that book one day—"*A Foreign Nurses guide to America*." Years later, the time has come. I give God the glory and praise

I was always in love with books. To this day, if my peers were to describe me I would be described as always seen reading a book.

I believed that there was a need for a foreign nurse to obtain a grasp of what nursing is like or can be like in America. The glitz, the glamour, the dread, the happiness, the wealth, the poverty may all be discovered. However, it starts with a decision. Maybe it will be help in their pursuit in their decisions to nurse in America. I hope this book would facilitate a foreign nurses' journey in American nursing. In an effort to educate foreign nurses I hope to accomplish enlightening other nurses as well.

My experience here has been extensive. I have learned in all walks of life. I have had life experiences, wake up calls, culture shock experiences. I have networked with networkers in the nursing and business industries. I have worked in nursing research and have travelled extensively in nursing. I have enjoyed the experience here in the USA.

Chapter Two

Make a Decision!

WRITING *A FOREIGN NURSE'S GUIDE To America* has given me the chance to vent slightly. One day, I may have to return to Caribbean. That is my heritage. I will pick up teaching and writing as a way to give back to my heritage. I think that my writing where I am can give me that start. The magic of "*the power of now*" (Eckhart Tolle) cannot be overly emphasize. In this phenomenal book, author Eckhart Tolle indicated that "time and mind are inseparable" (p. 48, Power of Now, 1999). We have to start with where we are and decide we plan to be. "Making a decision and act upon it." My 14-year-old son said to me one day, "Mom, make a decision and stick to it." I looked over at my son as I was driving, when he uttered those words to me, and reflected to myself: "That is it!" Wow!

I am proud of both of my children Sai and Harmonii. If were to be "childlike" and think the way children think we as adults can achieve so much. "Make a decision and stick to it!" (Harmonii, 2011) That was my 14-year-old son, Harmonii, told me. He does not know this, until he reads the book. From that day on, whenever I struggle it with choices of plans, I think back to: "Mom, make a decision and stick to it." I do not know if he heard this phrase somewhere or discovered quote he read somewhere, but it has become my guide in life now. Thanks, Harmonii, for your words of wisdom or sharing this statement with me. Thanks to my daughter Sai, a computer whiz, in her unique way.

When one makes a decision to relocate to the USA as a nurse, embrace that decision. Do not be here half-heartedly. America is one of the best nations to live. Vast amount of knowledge and experiences are available to anyone's advantage. When we arrive here, as nurses, we must remember to stick our mission and accomplish our goals, whatever they may be.

Chapter Three

Your past may be question

QUESTIONS HAVE BEEN ASKED OF foreign nurses regarding English has been learned to how arrival was made to America. I too have been personally have been asked questions about where I learned English, to how many languages I speak, how I get my nursing license—is there television there. Sometimes it may be asked naively. Other times, it often appears condescending. Times have changed. Several years ago it could have been the case. The universe appears to in and around us, thereby affecting the way in which we think and believe. was several years ago. There is a wide variety of commercial advertisement, along with the increase of travel and exposure to foreign nursing. There has been a greater understanding and adaptation to the nursing diversification and lifestyles. It may not be 100% understanding; however, it has gotten better.

Many foreign-trained nurses have had questions ranged from being funny, outrageous, and ignorant to plain insulting. To no fault of anyone, here is it is suffice to say ignorance is not really bliss. Do not take any negative or naïve comments personal. The advantage here is that as foreign nurses, we have the edge. In addition, we have to give respect to others, especially when residing in a different country.

I attended an accredited nursing school. I am a proud graduate and alumni of the school of nursing in St. Thomas, USVI. Information can be retrieved from the University of the Virgin Island's website. I completed the same NCLEX nursing exam offered here in the United States. There are two schools of nursing in the Virgin Islands, one in St. Croix, the other in St. Thomas. The nursing curriculum has the same syllabus as in the USA. The University of the Virgin Islands has two nursing programs, Associate Degree in Nursing, and Bachelor's Degree in nursing (n.d. UVI, 2011). The nursing program in St. Croix has a two-year nursing program. Residents from local neighboring islands, such as, St. Johns, Anne Garda, Virgin Gorda, and Tortola commute to St. Thomas and St. Croix in pursuit of the perspective nursing degrees.

Residents of Puerto Rico perform their nursing degree under the Republican State of Puerto Rico. Puerto Ricans and students who pursue nursing degrees perform their National Council Licensure Examination (NCLEX) exams in Spanish. For that reason, Puerto Rican nurses must retake NCLEX exams in English to be eligible to practice nursing in the mainland as well as the United States Virgin Islands.

I relocated to the United States mainland from St. Thomas, Virgin Islands as an Associate Degree registered nurse where I worked as an Emergency Department nurse. Here in the United States pursued a career in ED nursing as well. In addition, I have done travel nursing as well. I have learning has been extensive as nurse as well as socially, spiritually, and educationally as well.

In 1997, I was travelling to the Nevada, the thought came to me to write a foreign nurses guide to America. I believed that there was a need for foreign nurse to obtain a grasp of what nursing or the relocation experience may be like here nursing in America. Of course that experience is relative. The purpose of this books address issues that foreign nurses may encounter on their relocation here to the United States mainland. Some of the issues may be simple as well as being minor. The book is written in a light conversation piece. In addition, I hope that some of the questions that American nurses may have had may be addressed as well. However in hope of achieving some enlightenment, I trust that this book may serve as such a tool. I hope that may facilitate a foreign nurse's' journey in America. In general, nurses are well accepted in the work environment. However, many times foreign nurse may encounter changes or resistance if not well prepared. Being prepared puts a "foreign" nurse out in the forefront, thus decreasing any potential resentment, anxiety, or confusion.

Chapter Four

Differences in training identified

THERE ARE DIFFERENCES IN TRAINING found in many of the geographically trained IEN. The United States Nursing Boards determine who is qualified to work here based on the foreign nurse nursing curriculum and state board examination.

CARIBBEAN TRAINED NURSES:

Being from the Caribbean, I can relate more to that region best. Caribbean trained nurses, the majority are either trained under British or American nursing philosophy. Some are trained under French, Dutch, and, Spanish philosophies. The Caribbean is very much afro-eccentric, with some influence of African, Dutch, British, French, Portuguese, Arawak, Indian, and Caribe descent. However, nursing was influenced from Nightingale's theory and so was handed down from the London.

As we are we may be well are the Caribbean is comprised of British, Dutch, French, Spanish, and English-speaking islands. Each one of these islands has a health care system. Consequently, there are hospitals, nursing homes, and clinics on each island. Therefore, there are nursing schools as well. Some islands are ruled by different governmental system such as American systems, Dutch system, British system, and independent system. Some nurses relocate to London for training. If a nurse goes to an American accredited school system, that nurse takes the same NCLEX offered here in the United States mainland. Therefore, a United States trained-nurse from, St. Thomas, USVI who has successfully passed the NCLEX, USVI can apply for reciprocity to practice nursing in California, New York, and any other state in the United States, including Hawaii. Just as a Texas Nurse can apply for reciprocity can to practice nursing in Wyoming, the same applies. Nurses from the British islands, for example, Tortola, St. Kitts, Barbados, St. Lucia, Ghana, Philippines, India, and Canada all have different nursing laws to abide. The nursing curriculum is different in some aspects.

Many of these nurses went through the process of a nursing program, but the curriculum may be different. A nurse from the British islands, such as Anguilla, Antigua, or St. Kitts, go through a three-year nursing program to be a staff, nurse. Then additional one-two year is spent in labor and delivery where the nurse is trained to be a midwife. The staff nurses functions as a nurse practitioner would here in the United States to a certain degree in that she has been trained to suture and can suture simple wounds in the ED. A staff nurse has been successfully trained in pediatrics, med-surge, operating room, and recovery . . . basically all facets of nursing. The staff nurses have had extensive practical and classroom training prior to successful completion of the staff nurse exam. A foreign trained staff nurse is a registered nurse. Therefore, as mentioned a staff nurse is highly functional as a nurse practitioner here would in the US. In London, the same applies, with the nursing field; it goes from student nurse, to staff nurse to midwife to sister. There is also a matron that must be defined.

Because many of the foreign nurses went to London for training, it is important to go into any explanation of nursing in the United Kingdom.

In very recent, month, National Nursing day is established on May 6. Recently, I have asked a two-year American graduate-nurse, if she knows why nurse's day is celebrated on May 6. She did not know. National nurses' day is May six. May six is National Nurses Day. May 6th is the start of nurses' week and ends May 12 because of Florence Nightingale's birthday.

FLORENCE NIGHTINGALE

Florence Nightingale has been world renowned as the lady with the lamp. She is known as the pioneer of nursing because in the Crimean war. Born on May 12, 1820, Florence Nightingale has been known as the founder of modern nursing. Florence Nightingale was born in Italy to British parents. In 1859, Florence opening a nursing school, the Nightingale School for Nurses. In 1860, the official nurses training program commenced at the Nightingale School for nurses.

It is important to mention Florence Nightingale because of her early influence in nursing. Many nurses progress to adopt the British nursing philosophy

Mentioned has been made to Florence, because many British trained nurses developed Florence Nightingale's concept. Some nurses relocated to London to attend school there. Many nurses from Jamaica and Barbados also attended midwifery school in London. Attending a London trained school was considered reputable.

NURSING IN THE UNITED KINGDOM

Student Nurse - a new prospect has entered the nursing program and classroom and hands-on training is implemented.

Staff Nurse - a registered nurse who has completed three years of nursing in all areas, except midwifery.

Senior staff Nurse - a staff nurse who has successfully completed the midwifery program

Sister - a trained senior staff nurse who is usually in charge of a unit. She plans and implements appropriate nursing care.

Matron - the most senior nurse in the hospital in the united kingdom and other countries and islands as well, such as south Africa, Barbados, Jamaica, Nevis, Antigua, to name a few. The matron involves in the strategic operation of the hospital. She oversees nursing care and the nursing staff. She is most highly respected in the nursing field that operates with that capacity of nursing rank.

Philippine trained nurses: Just from association, a vast number of Philippine internationally educated nurses have migrated to the United States. I do not have the statistics on the percentage of IEN nurses are from the Philippines. If I were to make a calculated guess, I would estimate at least 50% of IEN in the USA, are from the Philippines.

Based on my interview with a few Philippine-trained nurses, they are mostly trained as BSN graduates. There is not a two-year or associate nurse program. Recently, there have been LPN trained nurses in the Philippines.

Chapter Five

Why nurse in America

SO, YOU WANT TO RELOCATE to America and practice nursing? It is important to be prepared. The goal is not to falter. "Internationally Educated nurses (IEN) are and continue to be an important part of the nursing workforce in the United States and throughout the world" (n.d. Transitioning Internationally Educated Nurses, OJIN, 2011). We as foreign nurses are a force to reckon in the health care industry. Any nurse is for that matter. However, is best that when a foreign nurse comes to America that he or she is a registered nurse qualified to practice nursing in the USA. As we can conclude, most nurses who relocate to the USA are already registered nurses in their country. Making the decision is the most difficult part. I wish to reiterate that as international nurses to never believe or be intimidated by the move. According to the an article written by the American Nurses Association posted in the *Online Journal of Issues in Nursing*(OJIN), the transition that IEN nurses faces is not because of lack of knowledge or skills (n.d. OJIN, 2011). I can attest to that. I acquired my RN license in St. Thomas, USVI. Over a decade ago when I recently relocated here, I was pulled (Neonatal Incentive Care Unit) NICU to work. There, a nurse asked if I collected the "TT". It was confused until I had to ask her what she meant. I thought it was lab test when it urine specimen she was referring. That is another issue one will encounter. Here in the USA many slangs and colloquiums are used in the health care work environment—something that many IEN nurses do not practice or may be unfamiliar. So be prepared to encounter that situation.

Chapter Six

USA Nursing Requirements

To PRACTICE NURSING IN THE USA one must have the qualifications of a United States trained registered nurse. In other words, a foreign trained registered nurse must be practice on the same curriculum as a United States practice nurse. I am putting registered nurses from the United States territories in the same category for reasons other than qualifications and accreditations. The reason as mentioned early, when coming from a different geographically region, we are all categorized as foreign nurses. To make it simply, nurse who have sat and successfully passed the US NCLEX do not need to retake any exams when relocating to the United States mainland. They simply have to apply for reciprocity and fill out the necessary application to apply for that state licensure. For example, a RN in St. John's USVI can apply to California State Board of nursing for her nurse license to practice in California. California state board will contact the USVI state board and verify completion and get the necessary documents for verification. That nurse has nothing else to do but wait for her process and send the application to receive her official license. Recently, licensures are no longer received in the mail. Verification can be made online. Some States in the past will bill a certificate of licensure acknowledging ones acceptance to practice nursing in the specific state. As foreign or international trained nurses, multiple state nurse licenses can be obtained at the same time.

Chapter Seven

Licensures—every nurse requires a license to practice nursing. Licensure must be current to be valid.

Holding one-two state nurse licenses

As FOREIGN OR INTERNATIONAL TRAINED nurses, multiple state nurse licenses can be obtained at the same time. IEN are trained in a vast variety of skills. Many foreign nurses are trained differently, thus giving the advantage of an edge over an American trained nurse. Reason being, a staff nurse in London, for example is qualified to insert and remove sutures. An advantage that many United States trained nurses may not have unless he or she is an advanced nurse practitioner.

WHEN IN ROME

Remember the cliché . . . when in Rome do as the Romans. Nurse practice acts mandates that nurse licensure are renewed every two years. Continuing education requirements must be made. In addition, Basic Life support (BCLS) is mandatory. Advanced credentialing is requirement based one's nursing profession, such as:

- ACLS (advanced cardiac life support)
- PALS (pediatric advanced cardiac life support)
- CEN (certified emergency nurse)
- CCRN (critical care registered nurse)
- TNCC (trauma nursing core course)

Know what is required is important to remain competitive and meet general requirements expected in the field. In other words, keep your Basic Cardiac Life Support (BCLS), ACLS, and nurse licensure are the basic requirements. No one has to tell to keep the basics current.

Chapter Eight

An honor to work in the USA

IT IS A PRIVILEGE AND an honor to work in the United States. Nurses are valued worldwide. America attractively advertises trained nurses sometimes question the reason International Educated Nurses (IEN) trained nurses come to America to work. Many nurses relocate for what they may think is a better way of life; some are curious; others are offered attractive packages; others are adventurous. More than two decades ago It has been advertised e since the in the late 1980's that there is a nursing shortage in the USA. Whether there is a shortage of nurses who are available or there is as nurse shortage supply, it is left for economists and healthcare administrators to decipher.

The issue at hand, once a decision is made to relocate know your why. Research the area that one plan to relocate. Decide if you can tolerate cold or hot weather conditions. Do an economic search.

Never talk negatively about America or its healthcare industry. If you have to, do not do it openly to offend anyone. Embrace where we are. When harnessed with feelings of homesickness or melancholy, make a trip to visit your homeland and family members, or find ways to embrace that feeling.

"By the year 2020, it is anticipated that a nationwide shortage of about 500,000 nurses" (n.d. PBS, 2010). IEN nurses can position themselves for nursing positions here in the US. It will become a situation of supply and demand. Because I am not an economist, I will not elaborate on the effect that it may have. However, foreign nurses can start planning and preparing for this impact to evolve.

Chapter Nine

Methods of US Training Available

AMERICA IS BY FAR ONE of the best nations that exists. There could be some setbacks upon relocation; there are also many advantages. The setbacks may include being away from one's family, lack of financial resources, language, cultural diversities, religion, and lack of friends. Know what one wants and decide upon it.

Most important, recognition must be made on the advanced education one can attain. The nursing opportunities in the USA are vast. These opportunities may include the attainment of the following:

- Advanced Registered nurse practitioner
- Physician Assistant
- Legal nurse consultant
- Independent Nurse contractors
- Certified Nurse Anesthetist

There are many international universities that have nursing programs, the University of Jamaica, the University of the Philippines, University of the Virgin Islands, to name a few.

As we are aware, there is a decline of nurse faculty members in the United States. According to an article written in the *Online Journal of Issues in Nursing, (*OJIN), nurse educators are on the decline (OJIN, 2011). Inadvertently, lack of a decrease in the nurse faculty members, the numbers will affect the supply of nurse graduates. Nursing students are finding it difficult to enroll in nursing schools here in the United States. The waiting list is long.

Phoenix online offers advanced degrees as well as nursing degrees online. These can be achieved in any parts of the globe. Visit their website for further information. There are many other online degreed and nursing programs available as well as at local universities and colleges

Kaplan University is listed as one of top names for online nursing degreed option. Kaplan University offers nursing programs online. It is an accredited school. Kaplan University "offers from diplomas to master's degree programs" (n.d. Kaplan university, 2011).

CGFNS is the Commission on Graduates of Foreign Nurses School. CGFNS testing is required based on one's nursing syllabus taken. Therefore, not all internationally trained nurses are required to take the CGFNS examination. When applying for reciprocity, some international trained nurses would be told if they have to take the CGFNS examinations. The CGFNS examination is required for some nurses not all. Please contact that office to find out the requirement. This examination "satisfies one of the immigration requirements for obtaining an occupational visa to work in the United States and is a prerequisite in some states for licensure" (Para1, CGFNS, 2006-2011). If one goes to the CGFNS website there is a guide to follow in obtaining certification.

Chapter 10

US Immigration

To work in the United States, an international nurse must have an occupational visa. Unless, you are a have US citizenship, obviously, one does not need a work visa. Some international nurses may have green cards and do not reside in the United States. They do not need occupational visas. However, please contact the United States immigration office about the regulations and working requirements for the details.

In the past, nurse recruiters were recruiting mass international nurses. Upon writing this book, less than a year ago, an immigration attorney said that the laws have changed. So please check with an immigration attorney or the immigration office to validate the requirements. In addition, the nurse recruiter at the United States' hospital should be able to advise one accordingly.

Chapter 11

Continuing Education

UNLIKE, MANY INTERNATIONAL NURSING MARKETS, here in the USA, a nurse is required to meet continuing education unites (CEUs). Random audits may be required by some nursing boards. The nurse is required then to submit his or her CEU's. Continuing education is important in staying abreast of one's nursing knowledge; it provides a professional advantage in the nursing industry. There are many continuing education departments to reference. Make sure that they are accredited. Most states offer CEUs as well. Thirty credits are usually required. Many continuing education offer free Ceu's. Some of my favorites cites are:

- American Nursing Association (ANA)
- Nursing Continuing Education (NCE)
- Medi-Smart
- American Nurses Credentialing Center (ANCC)

Additionally, one may have attained approved credits through courses such as advanced cardiac life support (ACLS), pediatric advanced life support (PALS), and trauma nurse (TNCC).

Chapter 12

Credentialing and Licensure Renewal

IN THE USA, THERE ARE various capacities of nurse practices. Here there are the following common ones:

- Licensed professional Nurses (LPNs)
- Licensed Vocational Nurses (LVNs) they are similar to LPNs.
- Advanced Registered Nurse Practitioners (ARNP)
- Nurse Midwives
- Legal Nurse Consultants (LNC)
- Certified Emergency Nurse (CEN)
- Critical Care Registered Nurse
- Certified Clinical Research Nurse
- Certified Nurse Operating Room(CNOR)

The important issue to be remembered that just about every department of nursing may have a certification. One may attain certification in that area usually with two or three years of nursing experience in that field.

There is a vast capacity of nursing practice here, from bariatric nursing to psychiatric nursing. Take your pick.

Licensure renewals are usually required every two years. License renewals are rather simple. It can be done online to the respective nursing board. In the past nurse state boards will mail one's updated licensed. No longer is that done. License verification is online. Usually a renewal reminder is done via mail. Renewals are done online. Mark sure that one CEU's are current.

Chapter 13

Wages and Scheduling

THERE ARE EIGHT-HOUR, 10-HOUR AND 12-hour shifts offered here. Some may work 16 hours. Upon average, most states offer 12-hour shifts. Differential pay is offered for evenings and night hours. Some States such as California, pay their nurses time and a half pay for working 12 hours after the first eight hours worked. For example, if a nurse works seven a.m.-seven p.m. After the first eight hours, the next four hours is paid at time and half. If work 16 hours, the first eight is paid at regular time, the second eight is paid at double time. In other states, the benefit advantage may not be offered. It is based on the labor code for that state. If you have a salaried position, one's time is calculated on straight salary paid-hours.

If a person works 12-hour shifts, the average work week may be forty-eight hours versus forty hours.

In your salary, FICA, and social security benefits are deducted from your salary. "FICA is a law that requires part of a worker's pay to be withheld for social security" (n.d.fica, 2011). There is no way around it.

Failure to meet these expectations may be encountered with the Internal Revenue Service. Every country has an IRS department.

Please have the employer explain how the IRS functions here for clarification. Some international markets do not pay internal revenue fees or claims the same way that it is done in the USA. Please check with a tax advisor and the IRS department.

Some States have different deductions in addition to others. Make sure the human resources depart explain that prior to started, so there are no surprises when one's final check is received.

Chapter 14

Education

As CITED EARLIER, MANY INTERNATIONAL nurses have BSN degrees; others have diplomas or two-year degrees. Here registered nurses have similar degrees. In addition, there are masters, advanced nurse degrees, PhD nurses, and doctoral nurses.

It is quite simple to advance one's degree once a nurse is an RN. Simply enroll in a local college or online colleges.

NCLEX is the national council licensure examination for registered nurses who used by the nursing boards to determine licensure decisions. (n.d. nclex, 2011). A graduate nurse must successfully pass the NCLEX exam for her to be granted the licensure to practice as a registered nurse.

Continuing education is required to stay abreast of current nursing practices. It is also required for licensure renewal.

Nursing education cannot be overly emphasized. No matter where one practices, nurses have to stay current.

Chapter 15

Nursing Shortage

AMERICAN NURSING COMPRISES OF A diverse nursing culture. Many nurses came here with dreams to be fulfilled. Many come because of the great nation that it is and would do anything to work here. Others have been solicited by nurse recruiters because of the nursing shortage.

There is a shortage of nurses in America. "The nursing shortage sweeping the United States may be worse than even the medical community is expected" (n.d. nursing shortage, 2011). The statistics are rising with the growing numbers of the anticipated positions that will be needed to be filled. This would definitely impact the healthcare system. Some foresee a health care crisis. Where America will obtain the nurses is left to be seen. With conflicts of decline in nursing faculty and the shortage of a nurse supply, America will have to turn somewhere to acquire registered nurses to work in its healthcare system.

It can be logically assumed that nurse recruiters will be looking at foreign markets such as Africa, Philippines, Caribbean, and Canada to supply its needs.

I am not an expert in nurse recruiting nor am I an economist, but as a fellow IEN I am enlightening foreign nurses to position for the potential crisis. If there were to be a health care crisis due to the supply of nurses, one implementation would be to recruit foreign nurses to supply the needs.

My position here is to facilitate an IEN in the decision to pursue a career in nursing in America as a foreign nurse. It is hoped for *A Foreign Nurse's Guide to America* will enlighten any foreign nurse with tips and options in facilitating that decision.

Thank God for the nursing career that we as nurses have chosen. The nursing profession is not an easy one. We are nurturers and provide compassionate care regardless of origin. The nursing career is a highly marketable. As nurse, one can position for work nationwide, once knowing the requirements. Many nurses went into the field because as nurturers, we are compassionate and caring for mankind. Many nurses are the head of household, and carry the financial burdens of their families. Nurses are highly respected in the field. It is a field that has mostly females in the profession. I am saying that to say, be shrewd in one's pursuit in one's journey as a foreign nurse in his or her nursing journey to America.

Examination one's decision and rectify if relocation is the best option. If so plan a time to fulfill your journey. Considerations should be given if one wishes to make America a permanent place of employment. With that in mind, one is focused on lifestyle one wishes to choose.

When relocating, consider the state of city one likes. Do not just take a position for high financial gains, only to find out it is very expensive to live there. In addition, make sure the offered position is a good fit. One that one can adjust culturally or to acclimatizes to that you. Those decisions will really benefit one's happiness and success in the position chosen. Review issues such as transportation, whether conditions, cost of living, salary scale, school, the chance for advancement.

If the ocean means is more important versus snow, consider places such as San Diego, instead of Colorado, or Wyoming. It may not matter, however. Do not settle for less because one is not from here. The options are vast.

Language is another important issue. English is the primary language here in America. If one is relocating from a Spanish culture or environment and may miss the Spanish language, consider a state with similarities.

Issues such as these may seem minor, but eventually, becomes missed. It also lessens the chances of being homesick much less.

Chapter 16

Language and Credit

SOME FOREIGN NURSES ARE REQUIRED to take English proficiency exams before authorized to work in the United States. When I graduated, from the CVI (College of the Virgin Islands) known now the University of the Virgin Islands (UVI), all graduates had to have successfully completed the English Proficiency Exam (EPE).

English is the universal language. English is spoken everywhere in the USA. Based on the influx of international residents, other languages have become rather prevalent. Spanish and Chinese have become common. In high schools, many students are fast learning Japanese, Chinese.

One may discover that English spoken in America is not the same to English spoken in London. When I speak English, I have been told that I speak "proper." There is much slang and used here that one has to become familiar.

I remember that I personally, had to get acquainted with some of the slangs or verbiage use when triaging or interview patients.

If English is not a person's first language, it is recommended to enroll in English classes. There are conversational languages one can learn via audio tapes. A well recommended one is *Rosetta Stone*.

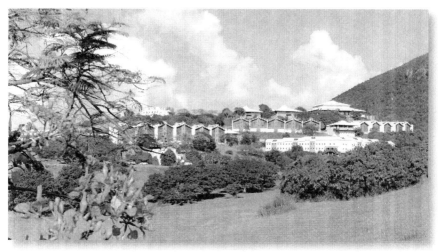

University of the Virgin Islands (UVI), St. Thomas Campus
(pic, UVI, EDU site, 2011)

**UVI has two campuses. One is on the beautiful island
of St. Thomas, Virgin Islands.**
The other campus is about 25 miles my air on the enchanting island
of St. Croix, Virgin Islands.

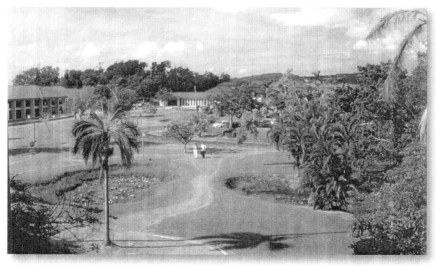

University of the Virgin Islands, St. Croix Campus (Pic, UVI, EDU, 2011)

The TOEFL is the test of English as a foreign language sometimes required of some foreign nurses from the nurse state board. I am uncertain who would need it. However, upon application of one's United States nurse licensure the requirements are made clear based one's original state licensure.

CREDIT SCORE

A good credit score is essential in America to survive the economic race. One either has to have a surplus of money or great credit. Either case have both is essential. If not, a good credit score helps one to succeed in America. Some people may differ with the comment, however, possessing a good credit score helps when making big purchases, such as a vehicle, a home, and a job. Some employers may look at one's credit score before hire that person.

According to the credit bureau, the credit score ranges from 300-850, 300 is bad and 850 is very good credit score rating (n.d. creditscorerange, 2011). A satisfactory credit rating helps qualify for mortgage loans, auto loans, employment, and making large purchases on credit.

When I first relocated to the USA, I had no credit. I neither had good nor bad credit. What I did was took out a bank loan and paid it off as quickly as I can. I also purchased a used vehicle—paid that off quickly and purchased a new vehicle soon after.

Information on credit is retrieved from the three financial bureaus, namely, Transunion, Experian, and Equifax.

It is my opinion that your credit score is very important. Please reference the one or all of the credit bureaus listed above for further elaboration.

Chapter 17

America's Health Care System

HEALTHCARE IN AMERICA IS FUNDED publicly, privately, and federally. America does not have a national health care system such as Canada or London. Residents and USA citizens can purchase private health care insurances themselves. Many private insurance entities, namely, to name a few, BlueCross Blue Shield, Aetna, and Mutual of Omaha sell insurance publicly and privately.

Privately-owned companies, including hospitals, offer insurance health care plans for employees. Most hospitals and other privately owned companies pay a percentage of the employees' insurance, with the employees paying the balance. Recently, the cost of private insurance has escalated and continues to be expensive. As a nurse, one can purchase family insurance plans through the privately own hospitals, or purchase health care plans independently. Whatever, the situation, the importance of health insurance coverage should not be overlooked.

In reference to work-related concerns, it is helpful to be aware of insurance coverage as well. In addition there is Medicare and Medicaid health insurance coverage.

Medicare covers health coverage for the disabled and United States citizens 65 and over.

Medicaid covers health insurance claims for low income families.

It is important to be aware of the American health care system. Information may be found on the websites, hospitals, and the library.

Chapter 18

Teachability and Credibility

TEACHABILITY

How teachable one is depends greatly on one's potential success rate. That finding was made by how Kevin Trudeau, one of most favorite author and coach. Trudeau indicated that before training or teaching someone on your team, to determine that person's teachability index. On a scale of one to 10, an eight would be acceptable. A score of 10 is an absolute indicator for chances of change and a chance to make a positive success. It is important to develop a high teachable score. In audio trainings that I have used through Kevin Trudeau, he said that for one to be teachable one must be coachable. The combination of both compounds of high teachablity and coachability indexes bring about success. Both indexes should be high to attain the possibility of a success rate. In so saying, develop a sense of urgency in coachability and teachability goals. Learn as much as one can. Build one's educational portfolio is important in a foreign nurses journey in America. Become an expert in the field one choses. Jim Rohn said in his book, *The Seasons of Life,* learn as much as you can be the most you can because "it is not the blowing of the wind but the set of the sail" (n.d. Jim Rohn, 2002).

Knowledge is not only power; it is most powerful on when and how it is used. Preparation cannot be overemphasized. Therefore, while being on a mission in America, for whatever one's purpose, obtaining advance degrees and credentials respected in one's field is crucial. Learn whatever you can. Attend training and continuing education.

CREDIBILITY

Nightingale was infamously known as the "lady with the lamp" (n.d. Nightingale, 2011). She gained credibility in her diligence as she took care of wounded soldiers. As nurses, we must gain respect in the nursing field by obtaining credibility.

Credibility may start from living a good quality life—one free from drugs and substance abuses. Credibility may also qualify a person's reliability and certified training achieved. On one's journey here, one may be exposed to nurses and health care workers who have abused narcotics and alcohol. Some of these nurses are treated on what is called a Training Program Accreditation Plan (TPAP). Where I come from, I never heard of any nurse who abused narcotics. Despite of a nurse's dilemma, one must try to and be empathetic and caring to nurses who have been treated for TPAP. One could lose one's nursing license for drug and substance abuse. Just be aware that it happens. Do what one can to safeguard one's dignity and safety for patients when administering narcotics.

As nurses, we have to work on ourselves. We have to take care of health, emotionally, spiritually, socially, and physically. Take time to love ourselves. Find the programs to embrace ourselves and others.

It is quite easy to lose credibility as a worker here in the USA. It may start as simple with one's credit report. Credit report as discuss

Chapter Nineteen

Nursing—a caring profession

NURSING IS A PROFESSION OF caring. No matter where one is trained, nurses are compassionate. The patients are the same; the philosophy is the same. Florence Nightingale's theory indicated just that: "Nursing is an art and a science" (n.d. Delmar). As one of the first nursing theorist, a nursing foreign, mentioned earlier, she to promote the conceptual concepts of the fundamental of nursing. There were other theorists who followed her work graciously, namely, Jean Watson, Dorethea Orem, Myra Levine, Sister Calista Roy, and Hildegard Peplau. The point is that these entire theorists came for all areas of the globe in essence to achieve a common goal—provide compassionate care implementing nursing fundamentals.

No matter where a nurse has traveled, a nurse's journey is committed one. A nurse's journey is one of commitment, nurture, compassion, and quest to meet the needs of human kind. A foreign nurse's journey is no different except when encountered by cultural differences, pain, trials, resistance, and diversities. However, nurses are strong, and have endurance. A quality we may be all made of. A foreign nurse's guide is a book to remind the foreign nurse of all those qualities that curtails us. A pride that we possess and are consistent.

In concluding, I hope that this book has served as enlightenment to a foreign nurse's guide to America. Many foreign nurses are prepared for the journey; some are not. Make the journey a successful one. America is one of the best Nation's that one can reside. The experiences are vast. Sometimes they experiences encountered can be horrendous; other times, the experiences are rewarding. In lieu of that the foreign nurse the experience can be a home away from home. One's stay here whether it is temporary or a lifetime can be a successful and happy one depends on the way it is planned. The choice and decisions made before and during one's stay in America is all relative to the choices one prepares for the start to the finish. As a foreign nurse, the journey to America is an eventful one. We can celebrate or successes and we venture to one of the most beautiful countries in the World, the United States of America!

Resources

- www.ana.com

- www.ancc.com

- www.cengage.com/country

- www.cgfns.com

- www.colormefine.com

- www.creditscores.com

- www.englishproficiencyexams.com

- www.elitewellmessproducts.com

- www.experian.com

- www.equifax.com

- www.legalnurseconsulting.com

- www.nclex.com

- www.nlnac.org

- www.nursing.com

- www.nursinglicencsure.com

- [www.usaaimmigration.com,](www.usaaimmigration.com)

- www.nursingstateboards.com

- www.salary.com

- www.sugarlandjuiceplus.com

- www.toefl.com

- www.transunion.com

References

Florence Nightingale. (2011). Retrieved from http://www.answers.com/topic/florence-nightingale

University of the Virgin Islands. (2008-2011). Retrieved from http://www.uvi.edu/sites/uvi/Pages/Programs-Home.aspx?s=VI

American Nurses Association, Inc. (2011). *Transitioning Internationally Educated Nurses for Success: A Model Program*. Retrieved from http://www.nursingworld.org/MainMenuCategories/ANAMarketplace/ANAPeriodicals/OJIN/TableofContents/vol132008/No2May08/TIENS.html

Nurses Needed. (2010). Retrieved from http://www.pbs.org/now/shows/442/index.html

Kaplan University. (2011). *Learning at Kaplan*. Retrieved from http://online.kaplanuniversity.edu/Pages/campus-online-learning.aspx

CGFNS. (2006-2011). *the Certification Program Process*. Retrieved from http://www.cgfns.org/sections/programs/cp/cpsteps.shtml

WiseGeek. (2003-2011). *What is FICA?* Retrieved from http://www.wisegeek.com/what-is-fica.htm

National Council of State Boards of Nursing. (2011). *NCLEX Examinations.* Retrieved from https://www.ncsbn.org/nclex.htm

Nursing Shortage. (2011). Retrieved from http://articles.cnn.com/keyword/nursing-shortage

Credit Scores Range. (2011). Retrieved from http://creditscoresrange.net/

Rohn, J. (2002). *The Seasons Of Life.* Southlake, Texas: Jim Rohn International.

Tolle, E. (1999). *The Power Of Now.* Novato, California: NAMASTE Publishing and NEW WORLD LIBARY Tolle, E. (1999). *The Power Of Now.* Novato, California: NAMASTE Publishing and NEW WORLD LIBARY.

Delmar Cengage Learning. (n.d). *Nursing Fundamentals: Caring & Clinical Decision Making.* Retrieved from http://www.delmarlearning.com/companions/content/0766838366/students/ch3/faq.asp

Gutterman, D. (1999). *Saint Kitts and Nevis Federation.* Retrieved from http://flagspot.net/flags/kn.html

WorldWide Flag Company. (2010). Retrieved from http://www.flagco.com/zoomsearch/search.php?zoom_sort=0&zoom_query=america&zoom_per_page=10&zoom_and=0

About the Author

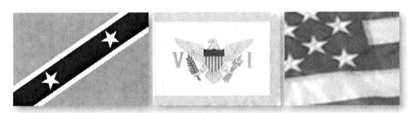

(Image by *Željko Heimer*, 01 Jan 2003, flagspot)
(n.d.worldwideflagcompany, 2010)

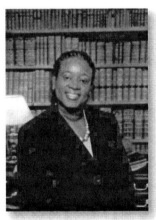

Shirley Lorraine Franks, RN, BS, MBA

"THE FOREIGN NURSE"

Faithful in our mission to pursue nursing in a foreign land!
On a journey of commitment!
Respected in the Field!
Enlighten by the experiences we learn!
Indispensable for the courage we possess!
Grateful for the opportunities received!
Nurturing . . . a quality we possess that we are called nice!

Shirley Lorraine Franks, RN, BS, MBA is daughter of Girlie Franks and Wentworth Franks, originally from the island of St. Kitts-Nevis. As an alumnus of the University of the Virgin Islands, she has also worked as a registered nurse in the US Virgin Islands.

Later, she relocated to the US mainland where she resides. She resides in Sugar land, Texas. Shirley has written this book a foreign nurse's guide to America—says that she has been a student of the late Jim Rohn. As a nurse, she believes this is the start of her writing career. She is a nurse and an entrepreneur with interests in health and beauty. Information can be received from cites listed in the resources page above.

She recognizes her school of nursing in the UVI as one of the best. To the nursing students at University of the Virgin Islands, she suggests that they are in a great place—learn it all and be good students.

Nursing is a compassionate and desirable profession. It gives the nursing vast opportunities to be explored.

With nursing, education is ongoing. The foreign nurse brings experience, education, culture and diversity to the American culture, a very unique quality indeed!

Famous quote by Author Jim Rohn: "I wish for you a life of wealth, health, and happiness; a life in which you give yourself the gift of patience, the virtue or reason, the value of knowledge, and the influence of faith in your own ability to dream about and to achieve worthy reward" (n. d. the seasons of life, 2002).

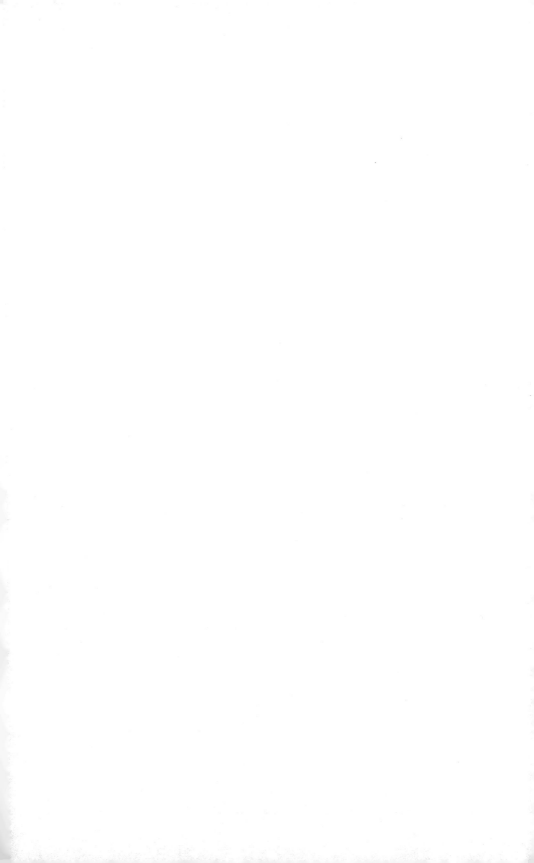

CPSIA information can be obtained at www.ICGtesting.com
Printed in the USA
LVOW08s2302110615

442154LV00001B/28/P